I0765764

Easy Keto Recipes Series

Keto Recipes for Breakfast

By Miranda Grey

ISBN: 9781695349346

TABLE OF CONTENTS

WHAT IS THE GOAL OF THIS COOKBOOK?

I prepared this recipe series so beginner keto practitioners such as yourself, can get the hang of preparing your own keto meals.

For the breakfast series, I have compiled easy breakfast meals for you to start creating in your own kitchen with some breakfast smoothie recipes to have your on-the-go options as well.

This book is for you if you're:

1. Just starting out in your keto journey.
2. On a keto diet for a while and don't want to figure out what to cook (Tired experimenting)
3. The type of person who prefers short-reads and not the overwhelming recipes by the hundreds (It's like being in a food court with too many shops to choose from)

This book is NOT for you if:

1. You're looking for fine-dining-and-cuisine-type recipes.
2. You're nitpicky and prefer books with calorie counts. You'll get a list of suggested apps and other resources in the last part of the book so be sure to make it.

In short, this will be your quick start guide to creating a healthy AND delicious combination of ingredients that won't destroy your taste buds and scar you or your loved one for life. My aim is to make your food preparation an enjoyable ordeal and not something to dread.

HOW TO USE THIS COOKBOOK...

There are 2 parts to this cookbook. Part One consist of proper recipes for breakfast (the most important meal of the day). Part Two consist of smoothie breakfast recipes for those who prefer it, people who are always on the go.

Good luck and happy eating!

PART ONE: KETO RECIPES FOR BREAKFAST

POWER BREAKFAST MUFFINS (KETO EDITION)

There are days when you don't have time to make breakfast. The best you can do is grab the nearest edible food you can find and make the most of it. For this reason, muffins have become a sort of staple for breakfast. The sad thing is most health experts agree that it's unwise to have muffins for breakfast, but that's partly because regular muffins are packed full of sugar and calories. Luckily with this recipe, you can have your cake (or, in this case, muffin) and eat it too.

Makes: 6-8

Prep Time: 10 Minutes

Cook Time: 15 Minutes

Total Time: 15 Minutes

Ingredients:

- 3 tablespoons plain Keto & Hot breakfast cereal
- 3 eggs
- 2 tablespoons heavy cream
- 2 tablespoons flaxseed meal
- 3 tablespoons coconut oil
- 2 tablespoons Erythritol
- 1 tsp. vanilla extract

- 1 tsp. baking powder

Method:

1. Preheat oven to 325 F

2. In a bowl mix Plain keto & Hot breakfast cereal, add coconut oil and mix well

3. Add the rest of ingredients and mix

4. Pour batter into 6-8 cupcakes and bake for 15-18 minutes

5. Remove and serve

Now you can eat your muffins early in the morning without worrying about packing some extra calories

GUILT-FREE ALMOND PANCAKES

Who doesn't like having pancakes for breakfast (or any time of the day for that matter)? One of the reasons they are popular is because they can easily be customized. Also, they are great on their own or combined with fruits. But did you know that the regular serving can have up to 227 calories? If you are watching your calorie intake, here's a recipe that substitutes regular flour with almond flour.

Makes: 4

Prep Time: 10 Minutes

Cook Time: 10 Minutes

Total Time: 20 Minutes

Ingredients:

- ½ cup almond flour
- 3 eggs
- ½ tsp. cinnamon
- 1 tablespoon butter
- ½ cup cream cheese

Method:

1. Place all ingredients in a bowl and mix using a blender

2. In a frying pan pour 2-3 tablespoons of pancake mixture and cook for 1-2 minutes per side

3. Remove and top with cinnamon or butter

You can also add your favorite berries or some chocolate chips.

CHEESY KETO SANDWICH

Sandwiches are another breakfast staple that's quick and easy to make. However, they can be chock full of carbohydrates, especially when you use white bread. A healthier alternative would be wheat bread because it is rich in fiber, which can aid in digestion and boost your metabolism.

Makes: 1

Prep Time: 5 Minutes

Cook Time: 5 Minutes

Total Time: 10 Minutes

Ingredients:

- 3 tablespoons shredded cheddar cheese
- 1 egg
- 1 slice bacon
- salt

Method:

1. In a skillet, cook half of the shredded cheese over medium heat and mold to a square as it is melting. Once melted, transfer on top of a slice of bread.

2. Cook the egg however you want and place it over the melted cheese and season with salt.
3. Slice bacon in half and fry until crisp. Place both halves on top of melted cheese and cooked egg.
4. Place the remaining cheese over the top and cover with the other slice of wheat bread.

Optional:

Grill the sandwich for a crunchy exterior and extra melty cheese

BACON BREAKFAST CUPS WITH GREEN SAUCE

Bacon is one one of the few ingredients that can be added to almost any dish and infinitely make it taste better. But did you know that you can also be creative with how you cook the bacon? This dish is a perfect example of serving bacon in a different way.

Makes: 3

Prep Time: 10 Minutes

Cook Time: 10 Minutes

Total Time: 20 Minutes

Ingredients:

- 1 cup baby spinach
- salt
- 1 cup parsley
- 4 garlic cloves
- 4 tablespoons hemp hearts
- 1 cup olive oil
- 4 slices bacon
- 1 cup arugula
- 1 egg
- 10 asparagus tips

Method:

1. To make the green sauce, mix arugula, olive oil, parsley, garlic cloves, baby spinach, hemp hearts in a blender and blend until smooth
2. Mold bacon slices into cups by forming them inside muffin tins (round baking molds would do as well). Cook bacon slices in the oven at 325 °F until slightly brown.
3. Beat the egg and combine with 3-4 asparagus tips and season with salt and pepper. Pour the egg mixture into each bacon cup and cook for another 12-15 minutes.
4. Remove bacon cups from muffin tin and transfer to plate. Pour over green sauce (or serve on the side).

MEATY AND CHEESY PEPPER RINGS

Red bell peppers are full of essential vitamins and minerals. They are rich in Vitamin A (good for the eyesight) and Vitamin C (boosts the immune system). Compared to green bell peppers, they are relatively sweeter in flavor. And they are much more tolerable compared to other spices because red bell peppers don't have capsaicin (the compound trigger that burning sensation on your tongue). No wonder is one of the go-to spices of most savory dishes.

Makes: 3

Prep Time: 10 Minutes

Cook Time: 10 Minutes

Total Time: 20 Minutes

Ingredients:

- 2 red bell peppers
- salt
- pepper
- 6 eggs
- 1 lb. breakfast sausage
- 3 tablespoons parmesan cheese
- coconut oil

Method:

1. Crush breakfast sausage into chunks.
2. In a skillet, brown the sausage and set aside once cooked.
3. Cut peppers into 4-6 rings and cook both sides on the skillet.
4. Pour the egg into the rings and add salt, some parmesan.
5. When ready, remove from the skillet and serve on the plate. Top the rings with some generous sprinkling of remaining parmesan.

ASSORTED CHEESE EGG BITES

Not all cheeses are made alike. Their taste and nutritional value changes depending on how they're processed. But because they are made from milk, they do have high calcium content, which is good for your bones. Plus, they add a creamy and smooth texture to any dish. This recipe contains swiss cheese (rich in B-12) and cottage cheese (packed with protein). If you craving some of that cheesy goodness but don't want to pack on the pounds, this dish is perfect for you.

Makes: 2

Prep Time: 10 Minutes

Cook Time: 20 Minutes

Total Time: 30 Minutes

Ingredients:

- 4 eggs
- ½ cup swiss cheese
- ½ cup fat cottage cheese
- ½ tsp. salt
- black pepper
- 2 thick slices of paleo sugar free bacon

Method:

1. Preheat oven to 325 F and place a baking dish

2. In a bowl mix cottage cheese, salt, pepper cheese, eggs and blend until smooth

3. Spray a muffin tin and pour the mixture into it, add chopped bacon and bake for 25 minutes

4. Remove and serve

HEARTY KETO BREAKFAST BOWL

The reason breakfast is regarded as the most important meal of the day is because it provides enough energy to help you start the day. For this reason, the ideal breakfast should contain the right amount of protein and carbs. Not only would these nutrients provide enough energy, but also kickstart your metabolism and aids in burning calories throughout the day. With that said, here is an easy but hearty breakfast recipe for you.

Makes: 1

Prep Time: 10 Minutes

Cook Time: 10 Minutes

Total Time: 20 Minutes

Ingredients:

- 2 eggs
- 2 strips bacon
- ½ up cheddar cheese
- ½ cup salsa
- 2 tablespoons butter
- ½ avocado

Method:

1. In a bowl scramble the eggs and place them into the skillet. Cook for 2-3 minutes
2. Top the eggs with shredded cheese and bacon
3. Slice avocado and place it over the bacon
4. Top with salsa and serve.

STIR-FRY VEGGIE BREAKFAST

There are mornings you still full from last night's dinner. You might think it's alright to skip breakfast when you feel that way, but at some point in the day you would feel the effects of it. Instead of skipping, you can just have a light breakfast. This recipe is just the solution to this conundrum.

Makes: 4

Prep Time: 10 Minutes

Cook Time: 10 Minutes

Total Time: 20 Minutes

Ingredients:

- 1 large turnip
- ½ paprika, garlic powder, salt
- parsley
- ½ onion
- 2 slices bacon
- 1 tablespoon olive oil

Method:

1. In a skillet, add the turnips and spices, cook for 5-6 minutes, add onion and cook for another 2-3 minutes
2. Chop the bacon and add to the skillet, cook for another 2-3 minutes.
3. Remove to a place and garnish with chopped parsley before serving.

MINI BREAKFAST MEATLOAFS

Despite its negative reputation in the health and medical industry, red meat is still regarded as a rich source of saturated fat, protein, zinc, and iron. So consuming pork and beef in moderation does have its benefits. And eating meat first thing in the morning is a good source of energy to kickstart your day.

Makes: 4

Prep Time: 10 Minutes

Cook Time: 10 Minutes

Total Time: 20 Minutes

Ingredients:

- 1 lb. pork sausage
- 1 egg
- 1 cup shredded cheddar cheese
- 4 slices bacon
- 4 slices ham

Method:

1. Preheat oven to 325 °F.

2. In a bowl, mix all ingredients

3. Divide mixture into 6-8 portions and pack into mini loaf pan with gaps in between.

4. Bake for 30 minutes, remove and serve. You could pair with your favorite bread or a side of eggs.

JALAPENO BREAKFAST MUFFINS

During those days you wake up groggy, sometimes a little spice is all you need to jolt you completely awake. Most peppers, like Jalapeno, are rich in capsaicin, a compound responsible for that burning sensation. However, this is also good for losing weight because it aids your metabolism. On top of that, they just add a bit some kick to any dish.

Makes: 4

Prep Time: 10 Minutes

Cook Time: 10 Minutes

Total Time: 20 Minutes

Ingredients:

- 8 eggs
- 8 oz. cheese
- ¾ cup heavy cream
- salt
- jalapeno
- 8 slices bacon

Method:

1. Preheat oven to 325 °F.
2. Slice bacon into chunks then distribute evenly in each muffin tin.
3. In a bowl, mix the ream, cheese, pepper, eggs and salt
4. Distribute into 8-10 muffin cups and top with jalapeno slices.
5. Bake for 15-20 minutes. When ready, remove from oven and serve.

Part Two: Smoothie Recipes for Breakfast

Keto Recipes for Breakfast

CREAMY MOCHA SMOOTHIE

Mornings wouldn't be complete without a mug of coffee. Most people drink this to help keep them awake throughout the day. But there are other benefits to coffee. For starters, it is rich in antioxidants (which slows down cell damage) and fiber (which aids in digestion). Studies also indicate that coffee drinkers have lower chances of heart disease, depression, and Alzheimer's disease.

Makes: 1

Prep Time: 5 Minutes

Cook Time: 5 Minutes

Total Time: 10 Minutes

Ingredients:

- 5 oz. cold coffee
- 3 oz. heavy cream
- 3 oz. almond milk
- 1 oz. sugar free chocolate syrup
- 1 oz. caramel syrup
- 1 tablespoon cocoa
- 12 oz. ice

Method:

1. In a blender, place all the ingredients and blend until smooth
2. Pour in a glass and serve (or store in the fridge and drink for later)

CHAI PUMPKIN SMOOTHIE

In recent years, Masala Chai has become all the rage. People were pleasantly surprised that they could mix spices with their favorite tea. But this beverage also has a wealth of benefits. It's been known to boost your immune system, alleviate nausea, and boost the health of your cells.   If you prefer a milder caffeine boost, this drink is for you.

Makes: 1

Prep Time: 5 Minutes

Cook Time: 5 Minutes

Total Time: 10 Minutes

Ingredients:

- ¾ cup coconut milk
- 2 tablespoon pumpkin puree
- 1 tablespoon MCT oil
- 1 tsp. chai tea
- 1 tsp. alcohol free vanilla
- ½ tsp. pumpkin pie spice
- ½ frozen avocado

Method:

1. Combine all ingredients in a blender and mix until smooth.
2. Pour in a glass and drink while still cold.

CASHEW MILK SMOOTHIE

These days, there are way more dairy substitutes for people who are lactose intolerant. The most popular would have to be soy milk, but other choices include almond and cashew milk. Surprisingly, they are just as creamy as regular milk but without the fat content. The best thing is these milks are quite easy to make.

Makes: 1

Prep Time: 5 Minutes

Cook Time: 5 Minutes

Total Time: 10 Minutes

Ingredients:

<u>Cashew milk</u>

- ¾ cup cashew nuts
- 4 cups water
- 1 tsp. vanilla extract
- ½ tsp. salt
- 1 tbsp. sugar (or your choice of sweetener)

<u>Smoothie</u>

- 1 cup cashew milk

- 1 tbsp. keto MCT oil
- 1 tbsp. keto nut butter
- 1 tsp. maca powder
- 1 handful ice

Method:

Cashew milk

1. Soak the cashew nuts in water overnight (or for four hours).
2. In a blender, combine all ingredients and blend on high for one minute.
3. If you prefer a smoother cashew milk, strain mixture in a cheese cloth and squeeze the milk out.

Smoothie

1. In a blender, place all the ingredients and blend until smooth.
2. Pour in a glass and serve or store in the fridge.

FRUITY COCONUT SMOOTHIE

It's amazing how much you can get out of a single coconut. From the water, to its milk, even down to the oil, almost everything is good for you. Coconut milk, in particular, can be used in a variety of ways. You can drink it straight or cook it in some curry. However it's consumed, it is definitely a rich source of vitamins and minerals.

Makes: 1

Prep Time: 5 Minutes

Cook Time: 5 Minutes

Total Time: 10 Minutes

Ingredients:

- ½ cup almond milk
- ½ cup coconut milk
- ½ coconut yoghurt
- ½ tsp. stevia
- 3 strawberries

Method:

1. In a blender, place all the ingredients and blend until smooth.
2. If you prefer a chunkier blend, leave out some strawberry chunks and only add once most of the drink is blended.
3. Pour in a glass and serve.

CREAMY SUMMER MILKSHAKE

Milkshake is probably the ultimate summer beverage. The fact that you could add just about anything in it and still tastes good, which makes it one of the most sought-after drinks. But if you are worried about how much calories you're taking, you can always substitute regular milk with almond or cashew milk.

Makes: 1

Prep Time: 5 Minutes

Cook Time: 5 Minutes

Total Time: 10 Minutes

Ingredients:

- 6 oz. plain almond milk
- 3 oz. crushed ice
- 1 oz. heavy whipping cream
- 1 oz. raspberries
- ¾ oz. sweetener of choice
- ½ oz. cream cheese

Method:

1. In a blender, place all the ingredients and blend until smooth or at least until ice has been completely crushed.
2. Pour in a glass and serve. You can also add a few more raspberries or some chocolate syrup for extra flavor.

CHOCO-AVOCADO MILKSHAKE

Avocado is another fruit that is becoming mainstream. It's not just used in guacamole anymore. And because it doesn't have an overpowering taste, it can be paired with almost anything. But more importantly, avocado is one of the most nutritious fruits. It's packed with vitamin K, C, B5, B6, and E. And because it's low in saturated fat, it's also good for your heart.

Makes: 1

Prep Time: 5 Minutes

Cook Time: 5 Minutes

Total Time: 10 Minutes

Ingredients:

- ½ avocado
- 2 tablespoons cocoa powder
- 2/3 cup coconut milk
- ½ cup crushed ice
- ½ cup water
- pinch of salt
- 1 tsp. lime juice
- stevia

Method:

1. In a blender place all the ingredients and blend until smooth
2. Pour in a glass and serve

COOL CHOCO COLLAGEN SMOOTHIE

The human body is comprised of many compounds with collagen being one of the most essential. It can be found on the tendons, ligaments, skin, and muscles. So if you want stronger bones, smoother skin, and toned muscles, you could do with some collagen.

Makes: 1

Prep Time: 5 Minutes

Cook Time: 5 Minutes

Total Time: 10 Minutes

Ingredients:

- 4 ice cubes
- ½ avocado
- 1 scoop keto chocolate collagen
- 1 tablespoon chia seeds
- 1 tablespoon almond butter
- ¾ cup heavy whipping cream
- 1 cup water

Method:

1. In a blender, place all the ingredients and blend until smooth

2. Pour in a glass and serve

FAT ALMOND BOMB SMOOTHIE

As mentioned earlier, there's plenty of other milk substitutes you can choose from one of which is almond milk. You can just buy this at the store; but if you want to put your own spin to it, you can make your own at home. It's relatively easy to make and won't cost you much.

Makes: 1

Prep Time: 5 Minutes

Cook Time: 5 Minutes

Total Time: 10 Minutes

Ingredients:

For the almond milk:

- 1 cup raw almonds
- 4 cups water
- 1 pinch salt
- 1 tsp. vanilla extract
- 1 pc. date

For the smoothie:

- 1 scoop collagen

- 1 tablespoon cacao powder
- 1 cup almond milk
- 1 cup ice
- 2.5 oz. avocado

Method:

For the almond milk:

1. Soak the almonds in water for at least 8 hours.
2. Drain the almonds.
3. In a blender, add the soaked almonds, water, date, vanilla, and salt and blend on high until thick and frothy.
4. Strain the almond chunks in a cheese to extract the milk.

For the smoothie:

1. In a blender, place all the ingredients and blend until smooth.
2. Pour in glass and serve.

CINNAMON PROTEIN SMOOTHIE

Out of all the spices, cinnamon is one of the few that's used for desserts, pastries, and other sweets. These days, there's plenty of cinnamon available in supermarkets. However, it was a rare commodity in ancient times and highly valued. So much so that it was presented as gifts for Pharaohs in Egypt. One of the reasons it is a highly-prized spice is because of its medicinal properties. If you're feeling a little under the weather, this smoothie might be the pickup you need.

Makes: 1

Prep Time: 5 Minutes

Cook Time: 5 Minutes

Total Time: 10 Minutes

Ingredients:

- ½ cup coconut milk
- ½ cup water
- 2 ice cubes
- 1 tablespoon coconut oil
- ½ tsp. cinnamon
- 1 tablespoon chia seeds
- ½ cup vanilla protein powder

Method:

1. In a blender place all the ingredients and blend until smooth.

2. Pour in a glass and serve.

FRUITY SUMMER SMOOTHIE

If you aren't a vegetable person, you could always rely on fruits for your daily dose of fiber. Not only are they good for you, but they taste good too. A lot of them are rich in Vitamin C, which is good for the immune system. Eating fruits on a daily basis also lowers your chances of bowel cancer and heart diseases.

Makes: 1

Prep Time: 5 Minutes

Cook Time: 5 Minutes

Total Time: 10 Minutes

Ingredients:

- ½ tsp. banana extract
- ½ tsp. blueberry extract
- ½ tsp. mango extract
- stevia
- 1 tablespoon oil
- ½ cup sour cream
- ice cubes
- ¾ cup coconut milk

Method:

1. In a blender place all the ingredients and blend until smooth Pour in a glass and serve

BONUS MATERIAL

Type the Link Below to Get Your Fee Guide Now!

http://bit.ly/YGAKS

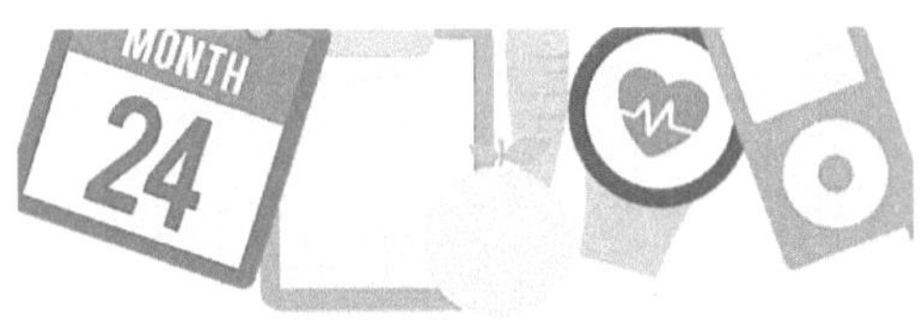

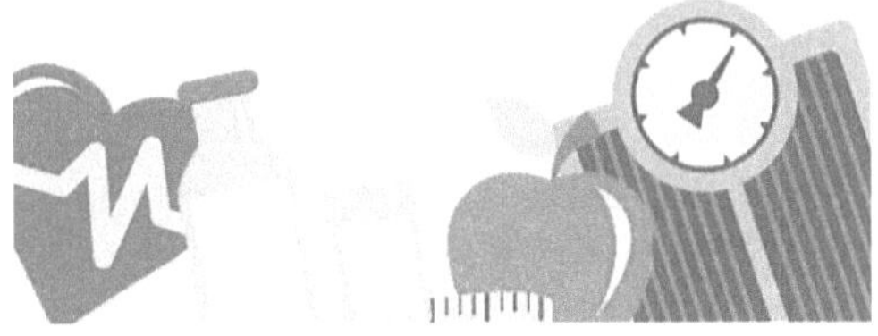

At first exposure on any type of diet, tracking is an important factor for you to be successful. As a thank you for just trying out the recipes in this book, you can get this free resource guide to help you achieve keto success!

ALSO FROM THIS AUTHOR

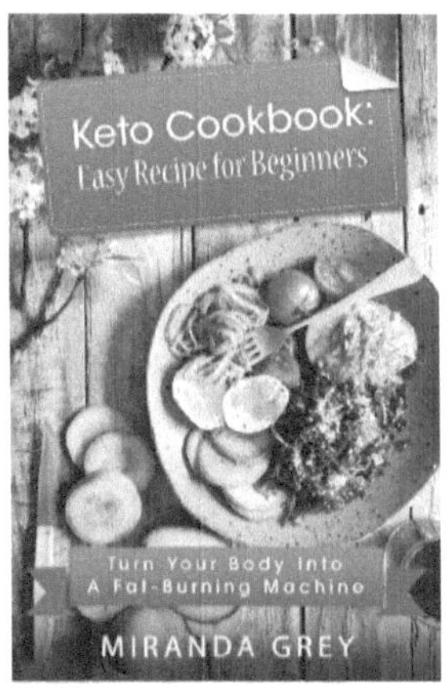

http://bit.ly/ketorecipesforbeginners

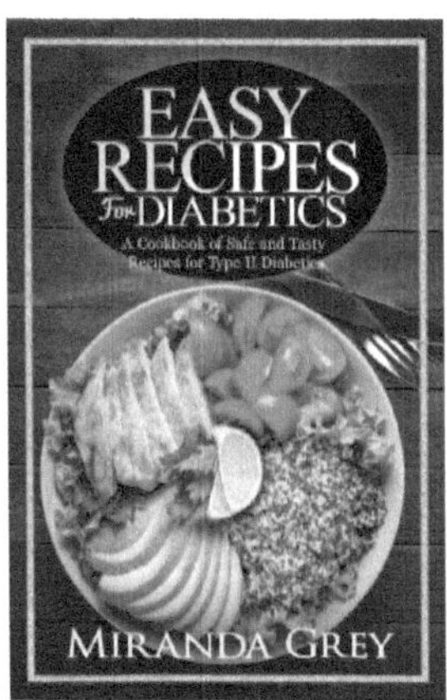

http://bit.ly/RecipesForDiabetics

ABOUT THE AUTHOR

Miranda Grey had always been the slim type ever since she was young so diet wasn't part of her vocabulary. Not until she gave birth anyway.

Because she had no experience with diet as a teenager, she had a hard time sticking to one and had experienced doing different types of diet and exercise that worked for a few months or so, but she would end up quitting because it left her tired and sore.

When she heard of the ketogenic diet, she went into a tailspin and followed every person she knew in social media who were under that diet and monitored their progress as well as research what she could about it.

Now, she is part of the growing movement of keto dieters that loves the benefits in both physical and mental. Plus the delicious food variations she could make with the allowed ingredients are numerous.